Fatty Liver Diet Cookbook for Seniors

Delicious, Easy-to-Prepare Dishes That Support Liver Health

Ennis James

Table of Contents

Introduction

Title: The Journey to Wellness: A Fatty Liver Diet Cookbook for Seniors

In a quaint bookstore nestled between bustling city streets, Emma found herself drawn to a display featuring a new cookbook titled The Journey to Wellness: A Fatty Liver Diet Cookbook for Seniors. As she leafed through its pages, Emma discovered more than just recipes; she found a guide that spoke directly to her needs and aspirations.

Emma had recently received a diagnosis of fatty liver disease. At seventy-three, she cherished her independence and zest for life, but the diagnosis had left her uncertain and apprehensive. The cookbook, adorned with vibrant images of wholesome meals and smiling seniors, promised more than just recipes. It offered a pathway to reclaiming control over her health.

The introduction captivated Emma with its clear explanations of the disease and the pivotal role of diet in managing it. She learned about the importance of nutrient-rich foods, low in saturated fats and sugars, to support liver function. Emma was relieved to find practical tips tailored specifically for seniors like her, ensuring she could adapt the recipes to fit her lifestyle and preferences.

Each section of the cookbook was thoughtfully curated, from hearty breakfast options like oatmeal with fresh berries to satisfying dinners such as grilled fish with roasted vegetables. The recipes were not just about nourishment; they were crafted to delight the senses and promote wellness. Emma could envision herself savoring a colorful quinoa salad or enjoying a comforting bowl of lentil soup, knowing she was nourishing her body in the best possible way.

But what truly convinced Emma to purchase the cookbook was its holistic approach. Beyond the recipes, it offered guidance on meal planning, shopping tips, and lifestyle adjustments. Emma realized that managing her condition wasn't just about what she ate, but also about embracing a balanced lifestyle that included regular physical activity and stress management.

As Emma stood at the bookstore counter, holding her newly purchased cookbook, she felt a renewed sense of optimism. She knew that this cookbook was more than just a collection of recipes; it was her companion on the journey to better health. With each turn of the page, Emma was reminded that age was no barrier to living well. Armed with knowledge and delicious recipes, she was ready to embark on her journey to wellness—one wholesome meal at a time.

And so, The Journey to Wellness: A Fatty Liver Diet Cookbook for Seniors became not just a book on Emma's shelf, but a beacon of hope and empowerment in her life.

This story illustrates how the cookbook serves as a valuable resource, providing practical guidance and encouragement to seniors like Emma who are navigating the challenges of managing fatty liver disease through diet and lifestyle changes.

Understanding Fatty Liver Disease

Understanding Fatty Liver Disease is crucial for seniors who are exploring ways to manage their health through dietary adjustments, as highlighted in the Fatty Liver Diet Cookbook for Seniors. Fatty liver disease encompasses a spectrum of conditions characterized by the accumulation of fat in liver cells. This buildup can lead to inflammation and liver damage over time, affecting its ability to function properly. Seniors, in particular, may be at higher risk due to factors such as age-related metabolic changes, sedentary lifestyles, and dietary habits.

The two main types of fatty liver disease are non-alcoholic fatty liver disease (NAFLD) and alcoholic fatty liver disease. NAFLD is more common and typically associated with obesity, insulin resistance, and metabolic syndrome. It can progress from simple fatty liver to non-alcoholic steatohepatitis (NASH), which involves inflammation and liver cell damage. Alcoholic fatty liver disease, on the other hand, is caused by excessive alcohol consumption and can also progress to more severe liver damage if alcohol intake is not reduced or eliminated.

Managing fatty liver disease revolves around lifestyle modifications, with diet playing a central role. The Fatty Liver Diet Cookbook for Seniors emphasizes the importance of a balanced diet rich in fruits, vegetables, whole grains, and lean proteins. These foods provide essential nutrients while reducing intake of saturated fats, refined sugars, and processed foods that can exacerbate liver inflammation and fat accumulation. Portion control and mindful eating are also encouraged to maintain a healthy weight and prevent further liver damage.

In addition to dietary changes, regular physical activity is essential for seniors with fatty liver disease. Exercise helps improve insulin sensitivity, reduce fat accumulation in the liver, and promote overall cardiovascular health. The cookbook offers practical tips for incorporating exercise into daily routines, taking into account mobility and fitness levels of older adults. Simple activities like walking, swimming, or gentle yoga can have significant benefits for liver health and overall well-being.

The progression of fatty liver disease can vary widely among individuals, making regular monitoring and medical supervision crucial. Seniors are encouraged to work closely with healthcare providers to manage their condition effectively. The cookbook provides insights into monitoring liver function through blood tests and imaging studies, helping seniors understand the significance of test results and their implications for dietary and lifestyle choices.

Beyond managing the physical aspects of fatty liver disease, the cookbook addresses the emotional and social aspects of living with a chronic condition. It emphasizes the importance of support networks, positive mindset, and self-care practices that contribute to overall health and quality of life. By fostering a holistic approach to wellness, the cookbook empowers seniors to take charge of their health journey and make informed decisions that promote liver health and longevity.

Ultimately, understanding fatty liver disease involves recognizing its complexities and tailoring management strategies to individual needs. The Fatty Liver Diet Cookbook for Seniors serves as a comprehensive guide, equipping seniors with knowledge, recipes, and practical advice to support their efforts in managing fatty liver disease effectively and improving their overall health outcomes.

Importance of Diet in Managing Fatty Liver

Managing fatty liver disease through diet is crucial for seniors seeking to maintain their health and quality of life. A fatty liver diet focuses on promoting liver health by reducing fat accumulation and supporting overall liver function. By adopting dietary strategies that prioritize nutrient-dense foods and minimize harmful fats and sugars, seniors can effectively manage their condition and potentially prevent its progression.

Central to a fatty liver diet is the emphasis on consuming foods that are rich in essential nutrients such as vitamins, minerals, and antioxidants. These nutrients play a vital role in supporting liver function and reducing inflammation, which are key factors in managing fatty liver disease. Seniors are encouraged to incorporate a variety of fruits, vegetables, whole grains, lean proteins, and healthy fats into their daily meals to ensure they receive a balanced intake of these beneficial nutrients.

In addition to nutrient density, the fatty liver diet focuses on moderating the intake of certain substances that can exacerbate liver damage. This includes reducing consumption of saturated fats, trans fats, and refined sugars, which are known to contribute to liver fat accumulation and inflammation. By making mindful choices about the types and quantities of fats and sugars consumed, seniors can help alleviate stress on their liver and support its healing process.

Furthermore, hydration plays a critical role in liver health as well. Seniors are encouraged to maintain adequate hydration by drinking plenty of water throughout the day. Proper hydration supports liver function by aiding in the elimination of toxins and waste products from the body, thereby reducing the burden on the liver and promoting overall detoxification.

The fatty liver diet also emphasizes the importance of portion control and mindful eating habits. Seniors are advised to eat smaller, more frequent meals to prevent overloading the liver with large amounts of food at once. This approach helps maintain stable blood sugar levels and reduces the likelihood of excessive fat storage in the liver, promoting better metabolic health and overall well-being.

Moreover, cooking methods are an essential consideration in the fatty liver diet. Seniors are encouraged to choose cooking methods that minimize the use of added fats and oils, such as baking, grilling, steaming, and sautéing with minimal oil. These cooking techniques help preserve the nutritional integrity of foods while reducing the intake of unhealthy fats that can contribute to liver damage.

Lastly, the fatty liver diet is not just about what seniors eat, but also about how they approach their dietary choices as part of a broader lifestyle strategy. Regular physical activity, stress management, adequate sleep, and avoiding alcohol are all important factors that complement a healthy diet in managing fatty liver disease. By adopting a holistic approach to health and wellness, seniors can optimize their liver function and enjoy a higher quality of life despite living with fatty liver disease.

Tips for Seniors Following a Fatty Liver Diet

Seniors facing the challenges of fatty liver disease can greatly benefit from adopting a tailored diet that supports liver health and overall well-being. When embarking on a fatty liver diet, it's essential for seniors to focus on consuming nutrient-rich foods while minimizing those that can exacerbate liver inflammation. Fresh fruits and vegetables should form the cornerstone of their diet, providing essential vitamins, minerals, and antioxidants that promote liver function and reduce oxidative stress. Additionally, seniors should incorporate whole grains like oats, brown rice, and quinoa, which offer fiber to aid digestion and help regulate blood sugar levels.

Lean sources of protein, such as poultry, fish, tofu, and legumes, are crucial for seniors following a fatty liver diet. These foods provide essential amino acids without the saturated fats found in red meats that can strain the liver. Seniors should opt for cooking methods that minimize added fats, such as grilling, baking, or steaming, to preserve the nutritional integrity of their meals. Healthy fats from sources like avocados, nuts, seeds, and olive oil should be included in moderation, as they provide essential fatty acids that support liver health and overall cardiovascular function.

Seniors should prioritize hydration by drinking an adequate amount of water throughout the day. Water helps flush toxins from the body and supports overall liver function. It's advisable to limit or avoid sugary beverages and alcohol, as both can contribute to liver inflammation and exacerbate fatty liver disease. Instead, seniors can opt for herbal teas or infused water to stay hydrated and add variety to their fluid intake.

Managing portion sizes is crucial for seniors following a fatty liver diet, as excess weight can exacerbate liver issues. By practicing mindful eating and listening to their body's hunger and fullness cues, seniors can maintain a healthy weight and reduce the burden on their liver. Regular physical activity is also essential, as it helps improve insulin sensitivity, promotes weight management, and enhances overall liver function. Activities such as walking, swimming, or gentle yoga can be beneficial and enjoyable for seniors looking to incorporate exercise into their daily routine.

Seniors should work closely with their healthcare provider or a registered dietitian to develop a personalized fatty liver diet plan that meets their individual nutritional needs and health goals. Regular monitoring of liver function through blood tests is crucial to assess progress and make necessary adjustments to the diet and lifestyle. Seniors should stay informed about the latest research and recommendations related to fatty liver disease management, as ongoing education empowers them to make informed decisions about their health.

In conclusion, following a fatty liver diet can significantly improve liver health and overall quality of life for seniors. By prioritizing nutrient-dense foods, lean proteins, healthy fats, hydration, portion control, and regular physical activity, seniors can effectively manage fatty liver disease and promote long-term wellness. With dedication, support from healthcare professionals, and a positive mindset, seniors can embrace the benefits of a tailored diet that supports liver health and enhances their overall well-being.

Chapter 1: Breakfast Recipes

Oatmeal with Fresh Berries

Ingredients:

1/2 cup old-fashioned oats
- 1 cup water or milk (almond milk or skim milk recommended)
- 1/2 cup fresh mixed berries (such as strawberries, blueberries, raspberries)
- 1 tablespoon honey or maple syrup (optional)
- 1 tablespoon chia seeds (optional)

Instructions:

1. In a small saucepan, bring the water or milk to a boil.
2. Stir in the oats and reduce heat to medium-low. Cook, stirring occasionally, for 5-7 minutes or until oats are tender and creamy.
3. Remove from heat and let it sit for 1-2 minutes.
4. Transfer oatmeal to a bowl and top with fresh berries.

5. Drizzle with honey or maple syrup if desired and sprinkle with chia seeds for added nutrition.

Nutritional Information (per serving):

- Calories: 250
- Total Fat: 4g
- Saturated Fat: 0.5g
- Cholesterol: 0mg
- Sodium: 20mg
- Total Carbohydrates: 48g
- Dietary Fiber: 7g
- Sugars: 10g
- Protein: 6g

Serving Size: 1 bowl

Cooking Time: 10 minutes

Whole Grain Toast with Avocado

Ingredients:

- 2 slices whole grain bread
- 1 ripe avocado
- Salt and pepper to taste
- Optional toppings: sliced tomatoes, a sprinkle of paprika

Instructions:

1. Toast the whole grain bread slices until golden brown.
2. While the bread is toasting, cut the avocado in half, remove the pit, and scoop out the flesh into a small bowl.
3. Mash the avocado with a fork until smooth, or leave it chunky if preferred.
4. Season the mashed avocado with salt and pepper to taste.
5. Spread the mashed avocado evenly onto the toasted bread slices.
6. Optional: Top with sliced tomatoes and a sprinkle of paprika for extra flavor and color.
7. Serve immediately and enjoy!

Nutritional Information:

- Calories: 250 kcal

- Total Fat: 15g
  - Saturated Fat: 2g
  - Trans Fat: 0g
- Cholesterol: 0mg
- Sodium: 300mg
- Total Carbohydrates: 25g
  - Dietary Fiber: 8g
  - Sugars: 2g
- Protein: 5g

Serving Size: 2 slices of prepared toast

Cooking Time: 10 minutes

Greek Yogurt with Chia Seeds and Fruit

Ingredients:

- 1 cup Greek yogurt
- 1 tablespoon chia seeds
- 1/2 cup mixed fresh berries (such as strawberries, blueberries, raspberries)
- 1 tablespoon honey or maple syrup (optional for sweetness)

Instructions:

1. In a bowl, combine Greek yogurt and chia seeds. Mix well.
2. Let the mixture sit for 5-10 minutes to allow the chia seeds to absorb some liquid and thicken.
3. Wash and prepare the mixed berries. If using larger berries, such as strawberries, slice them into smaller pieces.
4. Add the mixed berries on top of the Greek yogurt and chia seed mixture.
5. Drizzle with honey or maple syrup if desired for added sweetness.

Nutritional Information:

- Calories: 250 kcal
- Protein: 20g

- Carbohydrates: 30g
- Fat: 7g
- Fiber: 8g
- Sugar: 18g

Serving Size: 1 bowl

Cooking Time: 10 minutes

Spinach and Mushroom Omelette

Ingredients:

- 2 eggs
- 1/4 cup chopped spinach
- 1/4 cup sliced mushrooms
- 1 tablespoon diced onions
- Salt and pepper to taste
- 1 teaspoon olive oil

Instructions:

1. Heat olive oil in a non-stick skillet over medium heat.
2. Add onions and mushrooms, sauté until mushrooms are tender.
3. Add spinach and cook until wilted.
4. In a bowl, beat eggs with salt and pepper.
5. Pour eggs into the skillet, swirling to evenly distribute.
6. Cook until eggs are set, lifting edges to let uncooked eggs flow underneath.
7. Fold omelette in half and cook for another minute until fully cooked.
8. Serve hot.

Nutritional Information:

- Calories: 220
- Protein: 14g
- Carbohydrates: 4g
- Fat: 17g
- Fiber: 1g
- Sugar: 2g
- Sodium: 380mg

Serving Size: 1 omelette

Cooking Time: 10 minutes

Smoothie with Spinach, Kale, and Banana

Ingredients:

- 1 cup fresh spinach leaves
- 1 cup kale leaves, chopped
- 1 ripe banana, peeled and sliced
- 1/2 cup plain Greek yogurt
- 1 tablespoon chia seeds
- 1 tablespoon honey (optional)
- 1 cup almond milk (unsweetened)

Instructions:

1. Place spinach, kale, banana, Greek yogurt, chia seeds, and honey (if using) into a blender.
2. Pour almond milk over the ingredients.
3. Blend on high speed until smooth and creamy.
4. Pour into glasses and serve immediately.

Nutritional Information (per serving):

- Calories: 220 kcal
- Protein: 10g

- Carbohydrates: 35g
- Fiber: 7g
- Sugars: 18g
- Fat: 6g
- Saturated Fat: 1g
- Cholesterol: 5mg
- Sodium: 120mg
- Potassium: 670mg
- Calcium: 350mg
- Iron: 2mg

Serving Size: 1 smoothie

Cooking Time: 5 minutes

Quinoa Porridge with Almond Milk

Ingredients:

- 1/2 cup quinoa, rinsed
- 1 cup almond milk
- 1 tablespoon honey or maple syrup (optional)
- 1/2 teaspoon ground cinnamon
- Fresh berries or sliced fruit, for topping
- Nuts or seeds, for garnish (optional)

Instructions:

1. In a small saucepan, combine quinoa and almond milk. Bring to a boil over medium-high heat.
2. Reduce heat to low, cover, and simmer for about 15 minutes, or until quinoa is tender and most of the liquid is absorbed.
3. Stir in honey or maple syrup (if using) and ground cinnamon.
4. Remove from heat and let stand for a few minutes to thicken.
5. Serve warm, topped with fresh berries or sliced fruit, and garnish with nuts or seeds if desired.

Nutritional Information:

- Calories: 250
- Total Fat: 5g
- Saturated Fat: 0.5g
- Cholesterol: 0mg
- Sodium: 80mg
- Total Carbohydrates: 45g
- Dietary Fiber: 5g
- Total Sugars: 10g
- Protein: 7g

Serving Size: 1 bowl

Cooking Time: 20 minutes

Whole Wheat Pancakes with Berries

Ingredients:

- 1 cup whole wheat flour
- 1 tablespoon baking powder
- 1/4 teaspoon salt
- 1 cup unsweetened almond milk (or any milk of choice)
- 1 tablespoon honey or maple syrup
- 1 egg
- 1 tablespoon coconut oil (melted)
- 1 cup mixed berries (such as strawberries, blueberries, raspberries)

Instructions:

1. In a large bowl, whisk together the whole wheat flour, baking powder, and salt.
2. In another bowl, whisk together the almond milk, honey or maple syrup, egg, and melted coconut oil.
3. Pour the wet ingredients into the dry ingredients and stir until just combined. Do not overmix; a few lumps are okay.
4. Heat a non-stick skillet or griddle over medium heat. Lightly grease with coconut oil or cooking spray.
5. Pour 1/4 cup of batter onto the skillet for each pancake. Cook until bubbles form on the surface and the edges look set, about 2-3 minutes.

6. Flip the pancakes and cook for another 1-2 minutes until golden brown and cooked through.

7. Serve warm topped with mixed berries.

Nutritional Information (per serving):

- Calories: 250 kcal
- Total Fat: 8g
  - Saturated Fat: 5g
  - Trans Fat: 0g
- Cholesterol: 45mg
- Sodium: 350mg
- Total Carbohydrates: 40g
  - Dietary Fiber: 6g
  - Sugars: 10g
- Protein: 8g

Serving Size: Makes about 8 pancakes

Cooking Time: Approximately 20 minutes

Cottage Cheese with Pineapple

Ingredients:

- 1 cup low-fat cottage cheese
- 1 cup fresh pineapple chunks
- 1 tablespoon honey (optional)
- 1 tablespoon chopped nuts (optional, for garnish)

Instructions:

1. Place the cottage cheese in a bowl.
2. Add the fresh pineapple chunks to the cottage cheese.
3. Drizzle with honey if desired, for a touch of sweetness.
4. Sprinkle with chopped nuts for added crunch and flavor.
5. Mix gently to combine all ingredients.
6. Serve immediately and enjoy!

Nutritional Information:

- Calories: 250
- Protein: 18g
- Carbohydrates: 30g
- Fat: 7g
- Sodium: 350mg
- Fiber: 3g

Serving Size: 1 bowl

Cooking Time: 5 minutes

Scrambled Eggs with Vegetables

Ingredients:

- 2 large eggs
- 1/4 cup chopped bell peppers (any color)
- 1/4 cup chopped spinach
- 1 tablespoon chopped onions
- Salt and pepper to taste
- 1 teaspoon olive oil

Instructions:

1. In a bowl, whisk the eggs until well combined. Season with salt and pepper.
2. Heat olive oil in a non-stick skillet over medium heat.
3. Add chopped onions and bell peppers to the skillet. Sauté for 2-3 minutes until vegetables are tender.
4. Add chopped spinach to the skillet and cook for another 1-2 minutes until wilted.
5. Pour the whisked eggs over the vegetables in the skillet. Stir gently with a spatula to scramble the eggs and mix them with the vegetables.
6. Cook for 2-3 minutes, stirring occasionally, until the eggs are cooked through and no longer runny.

Nutritional Information: - Calories: 220 kcal

- Protein: 14g
- Carbohydrates: 6g
- Fat: 15g
- Fiber: 2g
- Sugar: 3g
- Sodium: 350mg

Serving Size: 1 serving

Cooking Time: 10 minutes

Muesli with Nuts and Seeds

Ingredients:

- 1 cup rolled oats
- 1/4 cup chopped almonds
- 1/4 cup chopped walnuts
- 2 tbsp sunflower seeds
- 2 tbsp pumpkin seeds
- 1/4 cup dried cranberries or raisins
- 1 tbsp chia seeds
- 1 1/2 cups unsweetened almond milk or low-fat milk
- Fresh berries or sliced fruit, for serving (optional)

Instructions:

1. In a large bowl, combine rolled oats, almonds, walnuts, sunflower seeds, pumpkin seeds, dried cranberries or raisins, and chia seeds.

2. Pour almond milk or low-fat milk over the oat mixture and stir well to combine. Cover and refrigerate overnight or for at least 2 hours to allow oats to soften and flavors to meld.

3. Before serving, stir the muesli and add more milk if desired to achieve desired consistency. Serve topped with fresh berries or sliced fruit, if using.

Nutritional Information:

- Calories: 350 kcal per serving
- Protein: 12g
- Carbohydrates: 40g
- Fat: 17g
- Fiber: 8g
- Sugar: 10g
- Sodium: 100mg

Serving Size: 1 bowl

Cooking Time: Overnight or 2 hours refrigeration

Chapter 2: Lunch Recipes

Grilled Chicken Salad with Olive Oil Dressing

Ingredients:

- 4 oz boneless, skinless chicken breast
- Mixed salad greens (lettuce, spinach, arugula, etc.)
- 1/4 cup cherry tomatoes, halved
- 1/4 cucumber, sliced
- 1/4 red onion, thinly sliced
- 1/4 avocado, sliced
- 1 tbsp olive oil
- 1 tbsp balsamic vinegar
- Salt and pepper to taste

Instructions:

1. Season the chicken breast with salt and pepper.
2. Grill the chicken breast until cooked through, about 5-7 minutes per side.

3. In a large bowl, combine the salad greens, cherry tomatoes, cucumber, red onion, and avocado.

4. In a small bowl, whisk together olive oil, balsamic vinegar, salt, and pepper to make the dressing.

5. Slice the grilled chicken breast and arrange it on top of the salad.

6. Drizzle the olive oil dressing over the salad and chicken.

7. Toss gently to combine and serve immediately.

Nutritional Information:

- Calories: 320 kcal
- Protein: 28g
- Carbohydrates: 10g
- Fat: 18g
- Sodium: 310mg
- Fiber: 4g

Serving Size: 1 salad

Cooking Time: 15 minutes

Lentil Soup with Vegetables

Ingredients:

- 1 cup dried lentils
- 4 cups vegetable broth
- 1 onion, chopped
- 2 carrots, diced
- 2 celery stalks, chopped
- 1 garlic clove, minced
- 1 teaspoon dried thyme
- Salt and pepper to taste

Instructions:

1. Rinse the lentils thoroughly under cold water.
2. In a large pot, sauté the onion, carrots, celery, and garlic until softened.
3. Add the lentils, vegetable broth, dried thyme, salt, and pepper.
4. Bring to a boil, then reduce heat and simmer for 30-40 minutes, or until lentils are tender.
5. Adjust seasoning if needed.
6. Serve hot, garnished with fresh herbs if desired.

Nutritional Information:

- Calories per serving: 250
- Total Fat: 1g
- Cholesterol: 0mg
- Sodium: 800mg
- Total Carbohydrates: 45g
- Dietary Fiber: 10g
- Sugars: 6g
- Protein: 15g

Serving Size: 1 cup

Cooking Time: 45 minutes

Tuna Salad on Whole Wheat Bread

Ingredients:

- 1 can (5 oz) tuna, drained
- 1/4 cup plain Greek yogurt
- 1/4 cup diced celery
- 2 tablespoons diced red onion
- 1 tablespoon chopped fresh parsley
- Salt and pepper to taste
- 4 slices whole wheat bread
- Lettuce leaves and tomato slices for garnish (optional)

Instructions:

1. In a mixing bowl, combine the drained tuna, Greek yogurt, celery, red onion, and parsley.
2. Season with salt and pepper to taste, mixing until well combined.
3. Toast the whole wheat bread slices until golden brown.
4. Divide the tuna salad evenly among two slices of toasted bread.
5. Top each with lettuce leaves and tomato slices if desired.
6. Cover with the remaining slices of toasted bread to form sandwiches.
7. Serve immediately or refrigerate for later.

Nutritional Information (per serving):

- Calories: 280 kcal
- Protein: 24g
- Carbohydrates: 27g
- Fiber: 5g
- Sugars: 4g
- Fat: 8g
- Saturated Fat: 1g
- Cholesterol: 30mg
- Sodium: 470mg
- Potassium: 320mg

Serving Size: 2 sandwiches

Cooking Time: 10 minutes

Quinoa Salad with Roasted Vegetables

Ingredients:

- 1 cup quinoa
- 2 cups water or vegetable broth
- 1 red bell pepper, chopped
- 1 yellow bell pepper, chopped
- 1 zucchini, diced
- 1 yellow squash, diced
- 1 small red onion, thinly sliced
- 2 tablespoons olive oil
- Salt and pepper to taste
- 1/4 cup fresh parsley, chopped
- 2 tablespoons balsamic vinegar
- 1/4 cup crumbled feta cheese (optional)

Instructions:

1. Preheat the oven to 400°F (200°C). Line a baking sheet
with parchment paper.

2. Rinse the quinoa under cold water to remove any
bitterness. In a medium saucepan, bring the water or
vegetable broth to a boil. Add the quinoa, reduce heat to
low, cover, and simmer for 15-20 minutes, or until the quinoa
is tender and the liquid is absorbed. Remove from heat and
let it sit covered for 5 minutes. Fluff with a fork.

3. Meanwhile, in a large bowl, toss the chopped bell peppers, zucchini, yellow squash, and red onion with olive oil, salt, and pepper. Spread the vegetables evenly on the prepared baking sheet.

4. Roast the vegetables in the preheated oven for 20-25 minutes, or until tender and slightly caramelized, stirring halfway through cooking.

5. In a small bowl, whisk together the balsamic vinegar and olive oil. Season with salt and pepper to taste.

6. In a large serving bowl, combine the cooked quinoa and roasted vegetables. Pour the balsamic dressing over the salad and toss gently to combine.

7. Sprinkle with chopped parsley and crumbled feta cheese if desired. Serve warm or chilled.

Nutritional Information (per serving):

- Calories: 280
- Total Fat: 10g
  - Saturated Fat: 2g
  - Trans Fat: 0g
- Cholesterol: 5mg
- Sodium: 280mg
- Total Carbohydrates: 38g
  - Dietary Fiber: 6g
  - Sugars: 4g
- Protein: 9g

Serving Size: 1 cup

Cooking Time: 45 minutes

Baked Salmon with Steamed Broccoli

Ingredients:

- 4 salmon fillets
- 1 lemon, sliced
- 2 cloves garlic, minced
- Salt and pepper to taste
- 1 tablespoon olive oil
- 4 cups broccoli florets

Instructions:

1. Preheat the oven to 400°F (200°C). Line a baking sheet with parchment paper.
2. Place the salmon fillets on the baking sheet. Season each fillet with minced garlic, salt, and pepper. Place lemon slices on top of each fillet.
3. Drizzle olive oil over the salmon.
4. Bake for 15-20 minutes, or until the salmon is cooked through and flakes easily with a fork.
5. While the salmon is baking, steam the broccoli florets until tender, about 5-7 minutes.
6. Serve the baked salmon with steamed broccoli on the side.

Nutritional Information:

- Calories: 300 kcal
- Protein: 30g
- Carbohydrates: 8g
- Fiber: 4g
- Sugars: 2g
- Fat: 16g
- Saturated Fat: 3g
- Cholesterol: 80mg
- Sodium: 150mg
- Potassium: 800mg

Serving Size: 1 salmon fillet with steamed broccoli

Cooking Time: 20-25 minutes

Turkey and Avocado Wrap

Ingredients:

- Whole wheat tortilla wrap
- 3 ounces of thinly sliced turkey breast
- 1/4 avocado, sliced
- 1/2 cup shredded lettuce
- 1/4 cup diced tomatoes
- 1 tablespoon Greek yogurt (optional)
- Salt and pepper to taste

Instructions:

1. Lay the tortilla wrap flat on a clean surface.
2. Spread Greek yogurt (if using) evenly over the tortilla.
3. Layer turkey slices, avocado slices, shredded lettuce, and diced tomatoes on top of the tortilla.
4. Season with salt and pepper to taste.
5. Roll up the tortilla tightly, folding in the sides as you go to create a wrap.
6. Cut the wrap in half diagonally for easier handling.

Nutritional Information:

- Calories: 280
- Total Fat: 11g

  - Saturated Fat: 2g
  - Trans Fat: 0g
- Cholesterol: 40mg
- Sodium: 550mg
- Total Carbohydrates: 26g
  - Dietary Fiber: 5g
  - Sugars: 2g
- Protein: 20g

Serving Size: 1 wrap

Cooking Time: 10 minutes

Bean Chili with Lean Ground Beef

Ingredients:

- 1 lb lean ground beef
- 1 onion, diced
- 2 cloves garlic, minced
- 1 bell pepper, diced
- 1 can (15 oz) kidney beans, drained and rinsed
- 1 can (15 oz) black beans, drained and rinsed
- 1 can (15 oz) diced tomatoes
- 1 cup low-sodium beef broth
- 2 tbsp tomato paste
- 1 tbsp chili powder
- 1 tsp cumin
- Salt and pepper to taste
- Optional toppings: shredded cheese, chopped cilantro, plain Greek yogurt

Instructions:

1. In a large pot or Dutch oven, brown the lean ground beef over medium heat until fully cooked. Drain any excess fat.
2. Add diced onion, minced garlic, and bell pepper to the pot. Cook for 3-4 minutes until vegetables are softened.
3. Stir in kidney beans, black beans, diced tomatoes, beef broth, tomato paste, chili powder, cumin, salt, and pepper.

4. Bring the chili to a boil, then reduce heat to low. Cover and simmer for 30-40 minutes, stirring occasionally, until flavors are well combined and chili has thickened to your desired consistency.

5. Adjust seasoning if needed. Serve hot, garnished with optional toppings like shredded cheese, chopped cilantro, or a dollop of plain Greek yogurt.

Nutritional Information (per serving):

- Calories: 320 kcal
- Protein: 27g
- Carbohydrates: 31g
- Fiber: 10g
- Sugars: 5g
- Fat: 10g
- Saturated Fat: 4g
- Cholesterol: 50mg
- Sodium: 600mg
- Potassium: 900mg

Serving Size: 1 cup

Cooking Time: 45 minutes

Whole Grain Pasta with Pesto and Cherry Tomatoes

Ingredients:

- 8 ounces whole grain pasta
- 1 cup cherry tomatoes, halved
- 2 cloves garlic, minced
- 1/4 cup pine nuts
- 2 cups fresh basil leaves
- 1/4 cup grated Parmesan cheese
- 1/4 cup extra virgin olive oil
- Salt and pepper to taste

Instructions:

1. Cook the whole grain pasta according to package instructions until al dente. Drain and set aside.
2. In a food processor, combine the garlic, pine nuts, basil leaves, and Parmesan cheese. Pulse until finely chopped.
3. With the food processor running, slowly pour in the olive oil until the pesto is smooth and well combined. Season with salt and pepper to taste.
4. In a large bowl, toss the cooked pasta with the pesto sauce until evenly coated.
5. Gently fold in the cherry tomatoes.

6. Serve warm, garnished with additional Parmesan cheese if desired.

Nutritional Information:

- Calories: 400
- Total Fat: 20g
  - Saturated Fat: 4g
  - Trans Fat: 0g
- Cholesterol: 5mg
- Sodium: 200mg
- Total Carbohydrates: 45g
  - Dietary Fiber: 7g
  - Sugars: 3g
- Protein: 12g

Serving Size: 1 cup

Cooking Time: 20 minutes

Veggie Burger on Whole Wheat Bun

Ingredients:

- 1 whole wheat burger bun
- 1 veggie burger patty (store-bought or homemade)
- 1 slice of tomato
- 1 slice of onion
- Lettuce leaves
- Mustard or ketchup (optional)

Instructions:

1. Toast the whole wheat burger bun lightly.
2. Cook the veggie burger patty according to package instructions or homemade recipe.
3. Place the cooked veggie burger patty on the bottom half of the bun.
4. Top with tomato slice, onion slice, and lettuce leaves.
5. Add mustard or ketchup if desired.
6. Cover with the top half of the bun and serve immediately.

Nutritional Information:

- Calories: 300 kcal
- Protein: 15g
- Carbohydrates: 45g

- Fiber: 8g
- Fat: 8g
- Saturated Fat: 1g
- Sodium: 600mg

Serving Size: 1 burger

Cooking Time: 15 minutes

Stir-Fried Tofu with Vegetables

Ingredients:

 - 1 block (14 oz) extra-firm tofu, drained and pressed
 - 2 cups mixed vegetables (bell peppers, broccoli, snap peas, carrots)
 - 2 cloves garlic, minced
 - 1 tablespoon grated ginger
 - 2 tablespoons low-sodium soy sauce
 - 1 tablespoon sesame oil
 - 1 tablespoon rice vinegar
 - 1 tablespoon cornstarch dissolved in 2 tablespoons water
 - 1 tablespoon olive oil
 - Salt and pepper to taste
 - Cooked brown rice, for serving

Instructions:

1. Cut the tofu into cubes and pat dry with paper towels.
2. Heat olive oil in a large skillet over medium-high heat. Add tofu cubes and cook until golden brown on all sides, about 5-7 minutes. Remove tofu from skillet and set aside.
3. In the same skillet, add garlic and ginger. Cook for 1 minute until fragrant.
4. Add mixed vegetables to the skillet and stir-fry for 3-4 minutes until they begin to soften.

5. Return tofu to the skillet. Add soy sauce, sesame oil, and rice vinegar. Stir well to combine.

6. Pour in the cornstarch mixture, stirring continuously until the sauce thickens and coats the tofu and vegetables evenly.

7. Season with salt and pepper to taste.

8. Serve stir-fried tofu and vegetables hot over cooked brown rice.

Nutritional Information:

- Calories: 320 kcal
- Protein: 18g
- Carbohydrates: 22g
- Fat: 18g
- Sodium: 580mg
- Fiber: 6g

Serving Size: 1/4 of recipe

Cooking Time: 30 minutes

Chapter 3: Dinner Recipes

Grilled Fish with Asparagus

Ingredients:

- 4 fillets of white fish (such as tilapia, cod, or halibut)
- 1 bunch of asparagus, trimmed
- 2 tablespoons olive oil
- 2 cloves garlic, minced
- Salt and pepper to taste
- Fresh lemon wedges for serving

Instructions:

1. Preheat the grill to medium-high heat.
2. In a small bowl, mix olive oil, minced garlic, salt, and pepper.
3. Brush both sides of the fish fillets and asparagus with the olive oil mixture.
4. Place fish fillets and asparagus on the grill. Cook fish for 4-5 minutes per side, or until fish flakes easily with a fork.

5. Grill asparagus for 3-4 minutes, turning occasionally, until tender and lightly charred.

6. Remove fish and asparagus from the grill. Serve hot with fresh lemon wedges.

Nutritional Information:

- Calories: 250 kcal
- Protein: 30g
- Carbohydrates: 5g
- Fat: 12g
- Fiber: 3g
- Sodium: 350mg

Serving Size: 1 fish fillet with asparagus

Cooking Time: 15-20 minutes

Chicken Stir-Fry with Brown Rice

Ingredients:

- 1 lb boneless, skinless chicken breasts, thinly sliced
- 2 cups cooked brown rice
- 1 cup broccoli florets
- 1 red bell pepper, thinly sliced
- 1 carrot, thinly sliced
- 1 cup snap peas
- 2 cloves garlic, minced
- 1 tbsp ginger, minced
- 2 tbsp low-sodium soy sauce
- 1 tbsp sesame oil
- 1 tbsp olive oil
- Salt and pepper to taste

Instructions:

1. Heat olive oil in a large skillet or wok over medium-high heat.

2. Add chicken slices and cook until browned and cooked through, about 5-7 minutes. Remove from skillet and set aside.

3. In the same skillet, add sesame oil and sauté garlic and ginger until fragrant, about 1 minute.

4. Add broccoli, bell pepper, carrot, and snap peas to the skillet. Cook, stirring frequently, until vegetables are tender-crisp, about 5 minutes.

5. Return chicken to the skillet. Add cooked brown rice and soy sauce. Stir well to combine and heat through, about 2-3 minutes.

6. Season with salt and pepper to taste.

7. Serve hot, garnished with chopped green onions or sesame seeds if desired.

Nutritional Information (per serving):

- Calories: 380
- Total Fat: 10g
  - Saturated Fat: 2g
- Cholesterol: 80mg
- Sodium: 500mg
- Total Carbohydrates: 38g
  - Dietary Fiber: 5g
  - Sugars: 3g
- Protein: 34g

Serving Size: 4 servings

Cooking Time: Approximately 30 minutes

Baked Cod with Roasted Vegetables

Ingredients:

- 4 cod fillets (6 oz each)
- 2 cups cherry tomatoes, halved
- 1 zucchini, sliced
- 1 yellow bell pepper, sliced
- 1 red onion, cut into wedges
- 2 tablespoons olive oil
- 2 cloves garlic, minced
- 1 teaspoon dried thyme
- Salt and pepper to taste
- Fresh parsley, chopped (for garnish)

Instructions:

1. Preheat the oven to 400°F (200°C).
2. In a large bowl, toss together cherry tomatoes, zucchini, bell pepper, red onion, olive oil, garlic, thyme, salt, and pepper until vegetables are evenly coated.
3. Spread the vegetables in a single layer on a baking sheet lined with parchment paper.
4. Bake for 15-20 minutes, stirring halfway through, until vegetables are tender and slightly caramelized.
5. While vegetables are roasting, season cod fillets with salt and pepper on both sides.

6. Remove the baking sheet from the oven and make space for the cod fillets among the roasted vegetables.

7. Place cod fillets on the baking sheet and return to the oven.

8. Bake for another 10-12 minutes, or until the cod is opaque and flakes easily with a fork.

9. Remove from oven and garnish with chopped parsley before serving.

Nutritional Information:

- Calories: 320 kcal per serving
- Protein: 35g
- Carbohydrates: 12g
- Fat: 15g
- Saturated Fat: 2g
- Cholesterol: 90mg
- Sodium: 320mg
- Fiber: 3g
- Sugar: 6g

Serving Size: 1 cod fillet with vegetables

Cooking Time: 30-35 minutes

Quinoa Stuffed Bell Peppers

Ingredients:

- 4 large bell peppers (any color)
- 1 cup quinoa, rinsed
- 1 ¾ cups vegetable broth
- 1 tablespoon olive oil
- 1 onion, finely chopped
- 2 cloves garlic, minced
- 1 zucchini, diced
- 1 cup cherry tomatoes, halved
- 1 teaspoon dried oregano
- 1 teaspoon dried basil
- Salt and pepper to taste
- ½ cup grated Parmesan cheese (optional, for garnish)

Instructions:

1. Preheat the oven to 375°F (190°C). Grease a baking dish with olive oil or cooking spray.

2. Cut the tops off the bell peppers and remove the seeds and membranes. Place them upright in the prepared baking dish.

3. In a medium saucepan, bring the vegetable broth to a boil. Add the quinoa, reduce heat to low, cover, and simmer for about 15 minutes, or until the quinoa is cooked and liquid is absorbed.

4. In a large skillet, heat olive oil over medium heat. Add chopped onion and cook until translucent, about 5 minutes. Add minced garlic and cook for another minute until fragrant.

5. Stir in diced zucchini, cherry tomatoes, dried oregano, dried basil, salt, and pepper. Cook for about 5-7 minutes, or until the vegetables are tender.

6. Remove from heat and stir in cooked quinoa until well combined. Adjust seasoning if needed.

7. Spoon the quinoa mixture evenly into the hollowed-out bell peppers. If desired, sprinkle grated Parmesan cheese on top of each stuffed pepper.

8. Cover the baking dish with foil and bake in the preheated oven for 25-30 minutes, or until the peppers are tender and the filling is heated through.

9. Remove from the oven and let cool slightly before serving.

Nutritional Information:

- Calories: 280 kcal

- Total Fat: 8g
  - Saturated Fat: 2g
  - Trans Fat: 0g
- Cholesterol: 5mg
- Sodium: 480mg
- Total Carbohydrates: 45g
  - Dietary Fiber: 7g
  - Sugars: 7g
- Protein: 10g

Serving Size: 1 stuffed bell pepper

Cooking Time: 45-50 minutes

Lean Beef and Vegetable Kebabs

Ingredients:

- 1 lb lean beef (such as sirloin or tenderloin), cut into 1-inch cubes
- 1 red bell pepper, cut into chunks
- 1 green bell pepper, cut into chunks
- 1 yellow onion, cut into chunks
- 8 cherry tomatoes
- 8 small mushrooms
- 2 tablespoons olive oil
- 2 cloves garlic, minced
- 1 tablespoon fresh lemon juice
- Salt and pepper to taste
- Wooden or metal skewers (if using wooden, soak them in water for 30 minutes before use)

Instructions:

1. In a bowl, combine olive oil, minced garlic, lemon juice, salt, and pepper. Mix well.
2. Add the beef cubes to the marinade, ensuring they are coated evenly. Cover and refrigerate for at least 30 minutes to marinate.
3. Preheat the grill or broiler to medium-high heat.

4. Thread marinated beef cubes, bell peppers, onion chunks, cherry tomatoes, and mushrooms onto skewers, alternating between ingredients.

5. Grill or broil the kebabs for 10-12 minutes, turning occasionally, until the beef is cooked to desired doneness and vegetables are tender.

6. Remove from heat and let rest for a few minutes before serving.

Nutritional Information:

- Per Serving (1 kebab, approximate):
  - Calories: 250 kcal
  - Protein: 25g
  - Carbohydrates: 10g
  - Fiber: 3g
  - Total Fat: 12g
  - Saturated Fat: 3g
  - Cholesterol: 60mg
  - Sodium: 350mg
  - Potassium: 600mg

Serving Size: 4 kebabs

Cooking Time: 30 minutes (including marinating time)

Turkey Meatballs with Whole Wheat Pasta

Ingredient:

- 1 pound lean ground turkey
- 1/2 cup whole wheat breadcrumbs
- 1/4 cup grated Parmesan cheese
- 1/4 cup finely chopped parsley
- 1 egg
- 2 cloves garlic, minced
- 1 teaspoon dried oregano
- Salt and pepper to taste
- 2 cups marinara sauce (low-sodium)
- 8 ounces whole wheat pasta
- 1 tablespoon olive oil

Instructions:

1. Preheat the oven to 375°F (190°C).
2. In a large bowl, combine the ground turkey, breadcrumbs, Parmesan cheese, parsley, egg, garlic, oregano, salt, and pepper. Mix until well combined.
3. Form the mixture into small meatballs, about 1 inch in diameter, and place them on a baking sheet lined with parchment paper.

4. Bake the meatballs in the preheated oven for 15-20 minutes, or until they are cooked through and lightly browned.

5. While the meatballs are baking, cook the whole wheat pasta according to the package instructions. Drain and set aside.

6. In a large skillet, heat the olive oil over medium heat. Add the marinara sauce and bring to a simmer.

7. Once the meatballs are cooked, add them to the marinara sauce and simmer for 5-10 minutes to allow the flavors to meld.

8. Serve the meatballs and sauce over the cooked whole wheat pasta.

Nutritional Information:

- Calories: 400 per serving
- Protein: 28g
- Carbohydrates: 45g
- Fat: 12g
- Fiber: 8g
- Sodium: 600mg

Serving Size:

- 4 servings

Cooking Time:

- Total: 40 minutes

Eggplant Parmesan with Marinara Sauce

Ingredients:

1 large eggplant, sliced into 1/4-inch rounds
1 cup whole wheat breadcrumbs
1/2 cup grated Parmesan cheese
1 tsp Italian seasoning
1/2 tsp garlic powder
2 large eggs, beaten
2 cups marinara sauce (low sodium)
1 cup shredded mozzarella cheese
2 tbsp olive oil
Salt and pepper to taste
Fresh basil for garnish

Instructions:

1. Preheat the oven to 375°F (190°C). Line a baking sheet with parchment paper.
2. Sprinkle eggplant slices with salt and let them sit for 15 minutes to draw out moisture. Pat dry with paper towels.
3. In a shallow bowl, combine whole wheat breadcrumbs, Parmesan cheese, Italian seasoning, and garlic powder.

4. Dip each eggplant slice in the beaten eggs, then coat with the breadcrumb mixture.
5. Heat olive oil in a large skillet over medium heat. Fry the breaded eggplant slices until golden brown, about 2-3 minutes per side. Transfer to the prepared baking sheet.
6. Bake the eggplant slices in the preheated oven for 20 minutes until tender.
7. Spread 1/2 cup of marinara sauce on the bottom of a baking dish. Arrange half of the eggplant slices over the sauce.
8. Top with 1 cup of marinara sauce and 1/2 cup of shredded mozzarella cheese.
9. Repeat with the remaining eggplant slices, marinara sauce, and mozzarella cheese.
10. Bake in the oven for 20-25 minutes until the cheese is melted and bubbly.
11. Garnish with fresh basil before serving.

Nutritional Information:

Calories: 250 per serving
Protein: 12g
Fat: 15g
Carbohydrates: 18g
Fiber: 5g
Sodium: 450mg

Serving Size:

4 servings

Cooking Time:

45 minutes

Stir-Fried Shrimp with Snow Peas

Ingredients:

- 1 pound large shrimp, peeled and deveined
- 2 cups snow peas, trimmed
- 1 tablespoon olive oil
- 2 cloves garlic, minced
- 1 tablespoon fresh ginger, minced
- 1/4 cup low-sodium soy sauce
- 2 tablespoons rice vinegar
- 1 teaspoon sesame oil
- 1 teaspoon cornstarch mixed with 2 tablespoons water
- 1/4 cup chopped green onions
- 1/4 teaspoon red pepper flakes (optional)

Instructions:

1. Heat olive oil in a large skillet or wok over medium-high heat.
2. Add minced garlic and ginger, sautéing until fragrant, about 1 minute.
3. Add shrimp to the skillet, cooking until pink and opaque, approximately 3-4 minutes.
4. Remove shrimp from the skillet and set aside.
5. Add snow peas to the skillet, cooking for 2-3 minutes until tender-crisp.

6. In a small bowl, mix soy sauce, rice vinegar, sesame oil, and cornstarch slurry.

7. Return shrimp to the skillet, pour in the sauce mixture, and toss to coat.

8. Cook for an additional 1-2 minutes until the sauce thickens and everything is well coated.

9. Sprinkle with chopped green onions and red pepper flakes if desired.

10. Serve hot.

Nutritional Information:

- Calorles: 210
- Protein: 28g
- Carbohydrates: 8g
- Fat: 7g
- Fiber: 2g
- Sodium: 500mg

Serving Size: 4 servings

Cooking Time: 15 minutes

Baked Chicken Breast with Sweet Potato

Ingredient:

- 2 boneless, skinless chicken breasts
- 2 medium sweet potatoes, peeled and cubed
- 1 tablespoon olive oil
- 1 teaspoon garlic powder
- 1 teaspoon paprika
- 1 teaspoon dried thyme
- Salt and pepper to taste
- Fresh parsley for garnish (optional)

Instructions:

1. Preheat the oven to 400°F (200°C).
2. Place the chicken breasts on a baking sheet lined with parchment paper.
3. In a small bowl, mix the garlic powder, paprika, thyme, salt, and pepper. Rub this spice mixture evenly over both sides of the chicken breasts.
4. In a separate bowl, toss the sweet potato cubes with olive oil, salt, and pepper until well coated.
5. Spread the sweet potatoes around the chicken breasts on the baking sheet.

6. Bake in the preheated oven for 25-30 minutes, or until the chicken is cooked through and reaches an internal temperature of 165°F (74°C), and the sweet potatoes are tender and slightly caramelized.

7. Remove from the oven and let the chicken rest for a few minutes before slicing.

8. Garnish with fresh parsley if desired and serve immediately.

Nutritional Information:

- Calories: 350 per serving
- Proteln: 30g
- Carbohydrates: 35g
- Fat: 10g
- Fiber: 6g
- Sodium: 250mg

Serving Size:

- 1 chicken breast and 1 cup of sweet potatoes

Cooking Time:

- 10 minutes preparation
- 25-30 minutes cooking

Veggie Stir-Fry with Tofu

Ingredients:

- 1 block (14 oz) firm tofu, drained and cubed
- 2 tablespoons olive oil
- 1 red bell pepper, sliced
- 1 yellow bell pepper, sliced
- 1 cup broccoli florets
- 1 cup snap peas
- 1 carrot, thinly sliced
- 3 cloves garlic, minced
- 1 tablespoon fresh ginger, grated
- 3 tablespoons low-sodium soy sauce
- 2 tablespoons rice vinegar
- 1 tablespoon sesame oil
- 1 tablespoon cornstarch mixed with 2 tablespoons water
- Cooked brown rice, for serving
- Sesame seeds and chopped green onions, for garnish

Instructions:

1. Heat 1 tablespoon of olive oil in a large skillet or wok over medium-high heat.
2. Add the cubed tofu and cook until golden brown on all sides, about 5-7 minutes. Remove from the skillet and set aside.

3. In the same skillet, add the remaining tablespoon of olive oil.
4. Add the garlic and ginger, and sauté for about 1 minute until fragrant.
5. Add the bell peppers, broccoli, snap peas, and carrot. Stir-fry for 5-7 minutes until the vegetables are tender-crisp.
6. Return the tofu to the skillet.
7. In a small bowl, mix the soy sauce, rice vinegar, and sesame oil. Pour over the tofu and vegetables.
8. Stir in the cornstarch mixture and cook for another 2-3 minutes until the sauce has thickened.
9. Serve the stir-fry over cooked brown rice, garnished with sesame seeds and chopped green onions.

Nutritional Information:

- Calories: 280 per serving
- Protein: 15g
- Carbohydrates: 20g
- Fat: 15g
- Fiber: 5g
- Sodium: 420mg

Serving Size:

- 4 servings

Cooking Time:

- 30 minutes

Chapter 4: Snack and Dessert

Healthy Snack Options

Greek Yogurt with Berries and Nuts

Ingredient:
1 cup Greek yogurt, 1/2 cup mixed berries, 1 tablespoon chopped nuts

Instructions:
Combine Greek yogurt with mixed berries and sprinkle with chopped nuts.

Nutritional Information:
Calories: 200, Protein: 12g, Fat: 8g, Carbohydrates: 18g

Serving Size: 1 cup

Cooking Time: 5 minutes

Hummus with Carrot and Cucumber Sticks

Ingredient:
1/2 cup hummus, 1 cup carrot sticks, 1 cup cucumber sticks

Instructions:
Serve hummus with carrot and cucumber sticks for dipping.

Nutritional Information:

Calories: 180, Protein: 6g, Fat: 8g, Carbohydrates: 20g

Serving Size: 1/2 cup hummus, 2 cups vegetable sticks

Cooking Time: 5 minutes

Apple Slices with Almond Butter

Ingredient:
1 medium apple, 2 tablespoons almond butter

Instructions:
Slice apple and serve with almond butter for dipping.

Nutritional Information:
Calories: 250, Protein: 5g, Fat: 16g, Carbohydrates: 26g

Serving Size: 1 medium apple, 2 tablespoons almond butter

Cooking Time: 5 minutes

Cottage Cheese with Pineapple

Ingredient:
1 cup cottage cheese, 1/2 cup pineapple chunks

Instructions:
Mix cottage cheese with pineapple chunks.

Nutritional Information:
Calories: 160, Protein: 14g, Fat: 5g, Carbohydrates: 16g

Serving Size: 1 cup cottage cheese, 1/2 cup pineapple

Cooking Time: 5 minutes

Conclusion

The "Fatty Liver Diet Cookbook for Seniors" stands as a vital resource for those seeking to manage their liver health through thoughtful dietary choices. This cookbook is meticulously designed to cater to the unique nutritional needs of seniors, providing not only a collection of delicious recipes but also a wealth of information to support overall well-being. By emphasizing the importance of nutrient-rich, low-fat, and low-sugar foods, this guide helps seniors make informed choices that promote liver health and reduce the risk of further complications.

Throughout the cookbook, seniors will find practical advice on how to incorporate wholesome ingredients into their daily meals. From hearty breakfasts to satisfying dinners, each recipe is crafted to be both flavorful and beneficial. The cookbook's focus on lean proteins, whole grains, fresh fruits, and vegetables ensures that seniors receive the essential nutrients they need without burdening their liver. Additionally, the inclusion of healthy snack and dessert options allows for indulgence without compromising dietary goals.

One of the standout features of this cookbook is its holistic approach to managing fatty liver disease. Beyond recipes, it offers valuable tips on meal planning, grocery shopping, and cooking techniques that minimize unhealthy fats and sugars. Seniors are empowered to take control of their diet and lifestyle, making choices that enhance their liver function and overall quality of life. The guide also emphasizes the importance of hydration, portion control, and regular physical activity, creating a comprehensive framework for healthy living.

Moreover, the "Fatty Liver Diet Cookbook for Seniors" recognizes the importance of personalization. Seniors are encouraged to work closely with healthcare professionals to tailor the dietary recommendations to their specific needs and health conditions. Regular monitoring and adjustments ensure that the diet remains effective and aligned with their health goals. This personalized approach not only addresses liver health but also supports other aspects of senior wellness, such as managing blood sugar levels, maintaining a healthy weight, and improving cardiovascular health.

In conclusion, the "Fatty Liver Diet Cookbook for Seniors" is more than just a collection of recipes; it is a guide to a healthier and more vibrant life. By following the advice and recipes within its pages, seniors can take proactive steps to manage their fatty liver disease and enhance their overall well-being. The cookbook provides the knowledge, tools, and inspiration needed to make lasting, positive changes in their diet and lifestyle. With dedication and the right resources, seniors can look forward to improved liver health and a greater sense of vitality.